PRAISE FOR *THE PALEOVEDIC DIET*

"Integrative medicine expert Dr. Akil Palanisamy makes both timeless knowledge and leading-edge research accessible in this groundbreaking and timely book. *The Paleovedic Diet* is rich with useful information on such diverse issues as gluten sensitivity, the human microbiome, detoxification in modern times and the rise of autoimmune disease. *The Paleovedic Diet* is a must-read for anyone serious about achieving optimal health and vitality."
—Andrew Weil, MD, world-renowned integrative medicine physician and bestselling author

"The Paleovedic Diet represents the best of integrative medicine, combining ancient wisdom with modern science and functional medicine to create a definitive roadmap to health. In an engaging and easy to read style, Dr. Akil presents the most up-to-date, evidence-based health information available today. He sheds light on topics such as optimal nutrition, the 100 trillion bacteria that make up your microbiome, the best way to exercise, and powerful detox practices. He reveals the hidden healing powers of spices and shows you how to use Ayurveda to customize a diet that's best for you. *The Paleovedic Diet* can help you lose weight, increase energy, and reverse disease."
—Mark Hyman, MD, eight-time #1 *New York Times*–bestselling author and functional medicine expert

"Dr. Akil deftly weaves the ancient wisdom of Ayurveda together with the principles of a nutrient-dense, Paleolithic diet to create a practical, individualized approach to wellness. If you've been looking for a way of eating and living that is tailored especially for your body and mind, this book is for you."
—Chris Kresser, LAc, *New York Times*–bestselling author of *The Paleo Cure*

"An impressively powerful intersection between East, West, and Ancestral Health. *The Paleovedic Diet* gives you a comprehensive guide to optimal health that integrates time-tested recommendations from ancient cultures along with the hard modern science that backs up their efficacy. Every page is chock full of invaluable, evidence-based guidelines on how to individualize your health plan for success. It's a truly impressive collection of information."
—Mark Sisson, *New York Times*–bestselling author of *The Primal Blueprint*

"In *The Paleovedic Diet*, Dr. Akil integrates his extensive clinical experience, the latest scientific research, and the most effective aspects of the Paleo diet with Ayurveda, the time-tested traditional medical system of India. He has created an enlightening, customizable, and easily actionable roadmap to optimal health that will open your eyes. *The Paleovedic Diet* has changed my approach to healthy living—and it'll change yours, too."
—Michelle Tam, *New York Times*–bestselling author of *Nom Nom Paleo: Food For Humans*

"*The Paleovedic Diet* is a powerful synthesis of the healing wisdom of a thousand years of ancient medicine and the precision and clear thinking of the best of scientific method. In elegant and easily accessible language, Dr. Akil Palanisamy makes available to us a wealth of previously unknown information about ourselves and the resolution of our most common problems. It is impossible to read this book without finding something in it that will heal you. A brilliant contribution to the health of every one of us."
—Rachel Naomi Remen, MD, *New York Times*–bestselling author of *Kitchen Table Wisdom* and *My Grandfather's Blessings*

"If you have been increasingly confused about what to eat, this is the book for you! Dr. Akil provides a sage and easy to follow middle way that blends the best of medical science with the wisdom of ancestral traditions."
—Victoria Maizes, MD, Executive Director, Arizona Center for Integrative Medicine

"Dr. Akil has beautifully blended the ancient, timeless wisdom of Ayurveda and Ayurvedic principles of healing with the light of modern medicine, integrated so that anyone can use it for his or her total healing."
—Vasant Lad, BAMS, internationally recognized Ayurvedic physician, author of *Ayurveda: Science of Self-Healing*

THE PALEOVEDIC DIET

A Complete Program to Burn Fat, Increase Energy, and Reverse Disease

Dr. Akil Palanisamy, M.D.

Foreword by Robb Wolf

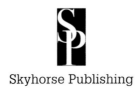

Skyhorse Publishing

Visit our website at www.skyhorsepublishing.com.

10 9 8 7 6 5 4 3 2 1

Library of Congress Cataloging-in-Publication Data is available on file.

Cover design by Laura Klynstra

Print ISBN: 978-1-63450-232-0
Ebook ISBN: 978-1-5107-0067-3

Printed in China

To my beloved wife, Aiswarya, and my beautiful daughter, Alisha—you have brought so much light, joy, and love into my life. You are everything to me.